For Clare, the most dedicated therapist I know.....

"The clearest way into the Universe is through a forest wilderness."

— John Muir

Introduction

I first thought about how rarely I see Monarda mentioned when I was writing my book *The Aromatherapy Bronchitis Treatment* and was addressing how wound healing problems in patients with emphysema seem *only* to be helped by essential oils. Thinking about oils containing the high levels of the thymol and geraniol required to bring about "the magic", I found the smallest mention of monarda, tucked away, hidden.

It was not the first time I had encountered the oil. I have used it myself in the past many times, and found its effects on catarrh to be wonderful. But it struck me...why wasn't anyone talking about it? Then I realised that, potentially, it may only be in the UK we don't know it so well, since it is not one of our indigenous plants. Likewise, its natural habitat doesn't lead it to references to the ancient Egyptians which we aromatherapy writers so love to use! Sure enough, on investigation, the beautiful flower is *deeply* ensconced in Native American Medicine.

The showy fragrant perennial almost verges on being a weed because it grows so prolifically in grasslands, and along the edges of streams, in North America. Statuesque plants, standing between 2-4 feet tall, they have long mint-like leaves (they are a member of a the mint family). Their shaggy flowers range from white, to pink, bright crimson or lavender purple depending on their species. It is a stunning plant with magnificent healing strength. I wanted to bring this to the attention of essential oil users who have not yet experienced its power.

Researching this paper has been a magical experience for me. I feel honoured to have found so much information about a medicine which to all intents and purposes would, until recently have remained hidden. I want to extend gratitude to all of the people who have contributed papers and information to this research. For anyone who wants to delve deeper there is a complete set of references at the end.

Table of Contents

Synonyms

Monarda is known by many names. It is often refered to as **Beebalm, Wild Bergamot, Goldmelisse** (German), **Heliaka ta pezhuta** (Dakota North American Indian), **Horsemint, Lavender wild-bergamot, Lemon mint, Lila temynta** (Swedish), **Monarda, Oswego tea, Pezhe pa** (Omaha and Ponca North American Indian), **Temynta** (Swedish), **Tsusahtu** (Pawnee North American Indian), **Wild bergamot, and Wild bergamot beebalm.**

History

The story of monarda is an entire lesson in American history and what the White Man found when he first placed his feet onto the new lands. Its Latin name was given in honour of Nicolas Monardes, a Spanish physician and botanist. Monardes was born in 1493, the year after Columbus first discovered America. His work into plant healing was to become some of the most important in history. In 1539 he discussed the importance of Greek and Arab medicine in *De Secanda Vena in pleuriti Inter Grecos et Arabes Concordia* . In 1540 *De Rosa et partibus eius* regales the virtues of both roses and citruses.

Then, most importantly, *Historia medicinal de las cosas que se traen de nuestras Indias Occidentales* described the plants and medicines found in the New World. Translated into

English by John Frampton *"Joyful Newes Out of the New Found Worlde"* gives us a fascinating insights into the indigenous species of the period.

In a moment we will look at how it was used by the various tribes across the plains. In order to grasp the beauty of the plant medicine, I feel it might be useful to imagine the culture of the time. The stereotypical picture we have in our minds of the Indians was of them riding fiercely on horseback but, in fact, horses were introduced by Spanish settlers in the 16th Century. Indian slaves had learned how to ride them when they were looking after ranches. Prior to that, no horses had been seen...and no wheels either.

The vast arid spaces between reservations, and the insular culture of many of the nations meant there would be little communications between them and yet the usage of monarda is constant and repeated across each of the peoples. Had they watched and seen how the plant changed the prognosis of disease, or did their wisdom and learning come from a different source?

We are familiar with the term Medicine Man or Woman, but in some ways it oversimplifies their role. Rather than being plant healers like you and I these sacred people were communicators with the Great Spirit.

In the Lakota tribe for instance Winyan wacan, is the "sacred woman" entrusted with locating healing plants and with remembering what their usage was for traditional medicine and symbolic usage. Her responsibility is to then pass along the information to her daughters. Winyan wacan is expected to receive powerful visions throughout her lifetime, and to eventually pass into and out of the spirit world at will. Could it be then, that ideas into plants healing potential were inspired, given perhaps in some type of vision? Many of tribes were nomadic, of course and so their wanderings may have offered some opportunities for information gathering.

Arwen Nuttal of The National Museum of the American Indian writes "The knowledge possessed by medicine people is privileged, and it often remains in particular families. Often enquiries about plant religious beliefs or practices from outside the tribe are viewed with suspicion." We are however lucky in the respect that Monarda fistulosa was known by the Pawnee by four specific names, based on their fragrance and so it is simple to track usage through early writings by settlers.

The different varieties of the plant were known as:

Tsuhata: Foul smelling

Tsotsu: No translation known

Tsakus Tawirat: Shot several times and still fighting

Parakaha: Sweet smelling

It is parakaha, that we now use as our essential oil *Monarda fistulosa*. There is also an essential oils relatively easily available *Monarda didyma* which is the version shown on the cover (because when else am I going to be able to have a hummingbird on the cover?!) *Fistulosa* by contrast is a lavender coloured flower which looks almost like a cross between the flower on a thistle and a lavender coloured Echinacea.

Monarda in Native American Medicine

I have collected together a list of the evidence I can find for each particular tribe and their medicine. These listings are for fistulosa because the chain of evidence is so much stronger. It amazes me how the usage can have been so similar when the chances to communicate its talents were so limited.

Blackfoot

The Niitsitapi, or Blackfoot Indians, reside in the Great Plains of Montana and the Canadian provinces of Alberta and Saskatchewan. This was a nomadic, hunter gatherer nation.

- Infusion of plant taken for coughs
- Poultice of a flower head applied to a burst boil and removed after the wound healed

- Poultice of plant pieces applied to cuts
- Infusion of plant taken for aching kidneys
- Infusion of plant and another plant taken and used as a steam to serve as an emetic
- Used to make a solution for sore eyes
- Root chewed for swollen neck glands
- Dried flowerheads used by invalids for sucking broth and soup

Cherokee

Originally, the Cherokee were located in the Southern Appalachian Mountains including the Carolinas, northern Georgia and Alabama, southwest Virginia and the Cumberland Basin of Tennessee and Kentucky. They were hunter-farmer nation, for the most part remaining in one place, close to their crops.

- Poultice of leaves used for headache
- Used for female obstructions
- Used as a carminative for colic and flatulence
- Poultice of leaves used for colds
- Used as a diuretic, diaphoretic and especially for "sweating off flu."
- Used as a carminative for colic, diuretic and diaphoretic

- Hot infusion of leaf used to "bring out measles" and infusion used as febrifuge.
- Infusion of leaf and plant top taken for weak bowels and stomach
- Infusion used for heart trouble
- Infusion of leaf or root taken orally and wiped on head for nosebleed
- Infusion of leaf used to "bring out measles" and infusion used to "sweat off flu."
- Used for hysterics and restful sleep.

Chippewa

The Chippewa Indians primarily inhabited the Northern regions of the United States. They could be found in Minnesota, Wisconsin, and Michigan

- Chewed leaves were placed in nostrils for headaches.
- Plant tops used for colds

Choctaw

Found in Oklahoma and Mississippi, with smaller groups found in Alabama, Louisiana and Texas

- Plant rubbed on child's chest for pain

- Infusion of leaves taken as a cathartic

Flathead

From western Montana, the Flathead reservation is home to the Bitterroot Salish, Kootenai, and Pend d'Oreilles Tribes

- Infusion taken for colds
- Plants hung on walls for colds
- Used for coughs
- Used to make a solution for sore eyes
- Infusion taken for fevers
- Infusion taken for flu and chills
- Infusion taken for pneumonia
- Used for toothache

Kootenai

- Infusion used for kidney problems

Koasati

Also known as Coushatta, the Koasati reservation lies just outside Louisiana

- Decoction of leaves used as a bath for chills

Menominee

Located in North Wisconsin

- Decoction of stem and leaves used as strengthening bath for infants
- Simple or compound infusion of leaves and flowers used as a universal remedy for catarrh

Meskwaki

The tribe has been historically located in the St. Lawrence River Valley, Michigan, in Wisconsin, Illinois, Missouri and in Iowa.

- Compound used for colds

Navajo

These were semi-nomadic hunter gatherers from Arizona, New Mexico, Utah and a small part of Colorado.

- Cold infusion of plant used as a wash for headaches

Ojibwa

Originally located around Lake Superior.

- Infusion of plant taken or used as a bath for infant convulsions
- Infusion of flowers taken for fevers
- Plant boiled and steam inhaled "to cure catarrh and bronchial affections."
- Decoction of root taken for "pain in the stomach and intestines."
- Infusion taken for stomach pains.

Sioux

The Sioux nation was largely nomadic following herds of bison across the plains. There were two main divisions of Sioux, Dakota and Lakota. They predominately lived in the northern Great Plains in lands that are today the states of North Dakota, South Dakota, Wisconsin, and Minnesota, but because of their nomadic nature might spend large amounts of time in other areas.

- Infusion of blossoms used for "hard cold."
- Infusion of blossoms used for fever.

Dakota Tribe

Also known as the **Santee,** *they lived on reservations Minnesota, Nebraska, South Dakota, North Dakota, and Canada.*

- Infusion of flowers and leaves taken for abdominal pains
- Decoction of flowers and leaves taken for abdominal pains

Lakota

Located in the Lower Mississippi region.

- Infusion of leaves used as a cough remedy.
- Infusion of leaves used on a cloth placed on sore eyes overnight.
- Poultice of chewed leaves applied to stop the flow of blood
- Infusion of leaves used for whooping cough
- Infusion of leaves used for fainting
- Leaves chewed while people were singing and dancing.

Crow

The Crow, who refer to themselves as **Afterpsáalooke** *in their own Siouan language historically lived in* *the Yellowstone River valley, which extends from present-day Wyoming, through Montana and into North Dakota. They had previously been part of the Sioux nations before breaking away in the early 1700's. They were a nomadic hunter gatherer nation.*

- Infusion taken for respiratory problems

Winnebago

*Also known as the **Ho-Chunk** originally native to the areas around Wisconsin, Minnesota, and parts of Iowa and Illinois*

- Decoction of leaves used on pimples and other skin eruptions on the face

I also found a reference to one of the Montana tribes using an:

- Infusion taken for expulsion of the afterbirth

But I cannot be more specific as to which one.

Its use in their everyday life

Blackfoot

The flowerheads of monarda were rubbed into unprepared hides to make them easier to clean.

According to alchemy-works.com, the Keres tribe would chew the leaves when they went out hunting. He suggests this could be connected with glamouring (shapeshifting and enticing). I can find no other supporting evidence for this. Just because it does not exist in the written word of course, does not mean it cannot be true. Monarda is most certainly a herb of transformation.

Cheyenne

Horses were rubbed down with flowers and leaves to perfume

them.

Plant matter was mixed with castoreum to make a heady hair oil. (Castoreum is the secreted from oil sac of a beaver; he uses it to mark his territory and ward off predators. It is deliciously musky scented and is a well sought after fragrance in contemporary perfumes, as well as being used as a food additive.)

By the 19th century it had become the traditional flower to give to brides to put into their bouquet. The flower would regulate their menses improving their fertility.

Throughout the nations we see a common theme of the leaves being also used as salads, as meat preservatives and also as teas.

It was this beverage that was to guarantee monarda's place in history. You may have noted that one of its synonyms was Ortega Tea. The plant (most likely to have been the scarlet *Monarda didyma*) grew lavishly around the Ortega region (which we now know as New York) and settlers took hints from the natives about the spicy beverage, and took to drinking Monarda as a tea. When the British (*I know, we have to poke our nose in everywhere don't we?*) imposed a tax on tea (*Camillea sinensis*), because of a surplus in the holds of The East India Trading Company, settlers turned to Ortega Tea as a bid to avoid the levy. When the "real" tea was thrown into the sea at the famous Boston Tea Party in 1773, most people had already converted their taste buds over to Monarda.

European Magickal uses of Monarda

By the 17th Century monarda had travelled across the seas and found herself in England. As such she is also found in Wiccan and Celtic magickal references.

Most popular seems to be that growing her in your garden will welcome the fae. There are also many references to how she attracts both money and love.

Spells using monarda

- Place fresh leaves in your purse and wallet to attract money
- Rub the leaves onto money to ensure it comes back to you
- Rub onto your hands before an interview or an important meeting
- Use it in spells to do with career success
- Run monarda into hot water to get rid of hexes, and to cleanse and invigorate
- Use in spells to attract love, for developing psychic intuition and for fertility
- To attract a partner soak the leaves in wine for several hours, then strain and share with a friend.

•

Ruling planet:

Mercury

(Again we have this connection with communication and co-ordination, one wonders if this might have been an alternate suggestion for chewing the leaves whilst hunting – mercury is of course, the archer!)

Mercury groups, organises and sorts things.

Physical Uses of Monarda Fistulosa

- Respiratory
- First line defence for acute infection. Use as soon as you get the tell tale sniffle or tickle
- Bronchitis
- Catarrh
- Coughs and Colds
- Colic and griping abdominal pains
- Aids and speeds digestion
- Constipation
- Headaches
- Wound healing
- Menstrual Problems
- Athlete's foot
- Anti bactericidal
- Strengthening and supportive
- Tonic to the liver and gallbladder.

The Emotions of Monarda

Energetically monarda is diffuse. Its strength is in movement and ridding the body and mind of stagnation. It is cleansing on physical, emotional and spiritual levels.

Those emotions that refuse to move on, which stagnate, fester and cause depression and of course disease, can be skilfully tackled using *Monarda fistulosa*. The jealousy that eats you up inside. The grief of loss. Nagging self doubt, that has nothing to do with your talents and potential and everything to do with your past. The fear which refuses to move out of the shadows...

Sustained pain of any description, all of these are monarda medicine.

I use the word *diffuse* because you can literally feel the energy diffusing, as if it relaxes the particles of negative emotions and lets them go. You can feel them lifting and opening up the chakras, raising your vibration, very quickly. This is extraordinary healing, in the very truest sense of the word, for patients whose ailments very clearly have an emotional or spiritual dimension.

In Dakota, *Monarda fistulosa* is referred to as *IleKaka ta pezhuta* which means Elk Medicine, and the spiritual aspects of the oil are very much aligned to their understanding of Elk spirit as a totem.

The elk are a strong and robust animal, whose stamina is marvelous. They do not reach their stride in life until well after puberty, and then adulthood comes quickly as the bulls antlers develop and fill out with their glorious velvet, almost overnight.

Opposed to conflict, the elk will avoid confrontation at all costs. But predators pick their fights carefully with this animal because he can fight long, hard and dirty. Stamina again, you see.

The elk is unusual because societally it is most interested in creatures of its own sex. Whilst females will cavort with males in the mating season, they are most happy with their mothers, aunts and their sisterhood. In fact, their very strength comes from their camaraderie, their kinship and their strength in numbers. Conversely, some may occasionally wander off and be perfectly happy on their own, then when the time is right they simply rejoin their herd again. Whilst one of their group is gone, the elk look after each other's young, drawing an inclusive protective bond around the whole tribe.

Native Americans value silence in a very different way to the way we tend to do so. Words are a profound teaching power.

They do not speak and chat in the way that we do. If a member of a tribe feels sad or angry, they will go off on their own to let the feelings pass. They will not speak. Where, in *our* society we might consider this behaviour in one of our own to be aloof, or concerning, they simply await for the time when they are ready to come back and socialise again. Their respect of their member's time alone is their own support mechanism.

Elk medicine teaches of the importance of turning to the sisterhood for support, but also being ready to value one's time alone. (I should actually say, turning to one's own *gender,* since the medicine works in the same way for men).

Again the spiritual aspect of monarda echos the physical attributes of the elk. It teaches us to pace ourselves for the long haul. To change our speed and approach in response to the terrain we see before us, in order to garner the strength to endure the toughest of challenges. And when the time comes to fight your corner...to dig in and give it all you've got.

Elk Medicine fights for what it believes in...long, hard, and usually successfully.

I like to think of that medicine surrounding the newborn menominee in his bathwater, only moments from drawing his first breath. Protecting strengthening...patiently growing.

The Spiritual Aspects of Monarda

This is a plant used in two of many of the plains tribes' most sacred rituals, the Sun Dance and the Sweat Lodge. The sun dance is performed around a cotton pole, and follows a full 28 days of cleansing rituals many of these in the sweat lodge, a willow hut, insulated and covered with hides and blankets. In the centre of the lodge are lava stones, and plants are thrown onto heated rocks to release their healing oils. Throughout the ceremony prayers, meditations and songs are sung to cleanse and connect with the Great Spirit.

The name for the ritual of the sweat lodge, *oenikika*, means the breath of life. William J. Walk Sacred, a Cree medicine man: explains "When you come out of a purification lodge, you don't feel the same as when you come out of a sauna. The ceremony is a rebirthing process. There's something that happens in a spiritual sense that is powerful and uplifting." He describes how the process of rebirth should be considered to be like a marriage ceremony conducted with one's self.

The rituals of the sweat lodge and the Sun Dance are of transformation; for moving forward.

The flower essence workers shine a radiant light on the vibration of Monarda. Capturing the essence by leaving the flowers to steep in water, rather than distilling it, their essence works more on the intuitive level, but has the same properties of an essential oil.

Dianne and John Pepper have written a beautiful page about monarda on their website Tree Frog Farm. They sell a flower essence, rather than an essential oil from the plant which has been grown with gemstones between the plants.

They connect the motto:

"I am the spiritual light piercing the collective consciousness to raise the frequency of your bodymind".

This is a glorious explanation of how monarda seems to remove old scripts, on a personal level, but on a far wider, more universal scale too. If you struggle to assimilate newer truths like how the emotions affect disease, or how abundance is everywhere, or even to feel your place in the universe as a whole...then monarda medicine is for you. Consider it like a crash course when you missed several weeks' lessons!

Aelena Charlotte Daemon speaks of how monarda *"Helps to accept more nourishing thoughts and beliefs. Feeling enthused and motivated to support dreams and goals that are of great value to you, even though others are not supportive or tell you that it "could never happen".*

And yes, that makes sense to me, because it does make you feel like you are almost floating above obstacles and hurdles. The biggest of that is always...the past. Of course, what are the most effective things you can do when your support system starts to cave?

- Look inside of yourself for reassurance and extra strength (rather than turning against the cynics)
- Draw a new supportive tribe to you.

Elk Medicine

Empowerment through the Goddess

Native American healing.

Wiccan healing.

Plant consciousness....magic.

I think where oils like rosemary and tangerine have that sharp kick that almost sticks a finger up at other people and says "I'll show you", monarda is more about "They are entitled to their opinion. Mine is different, that's all."

Mellow, reasonable, but very open minded.

Monarda's nervine qualities are lifting and opening. It promotes a sense of euphoria, of joy and of calm. The Lakota would chew the leaves whilst singing and dancing.

But this lifting, of course, is not for everyone. It is **so-oo-oo** feminine. Girlie-girl power. It is deliciously yin medicine, but for those who are not grounded, and already have their heads in the clouds, this medicine is almost dangerously stratospheric. In her stunning work, Kiva Rose of Bear Medicine Woman describes the problem of those not well enough grounded, "floating away on butterfly wings". Exquisitely put.

(For those who have read my book The Professional Stress Solution and have studied Yin medicine, monarda is Yin + to the power of ten!)

Clearly, she is a nicer person than me. I'm going to say: for some people, (and you know the type – the world owes them a living and everything is just beautiful, *d-ah-ling*) monarda is a recipe for candy-floss brains. (Translation for my transatlantic friends - cotton candy).

It's a fabulously happy oil though, which is what I like about it. Well, it would have to be, smelling like a citrusy bergamot wouldn't it? But more than that. Where most of the respiratory oils are clinical and a bit no nonsense really, monarda is light, beguiling, floaty. Its energy makes you smile and see magic and sweetness in the every day. Perhaps too, this is Elk Medicine, *let it go*, because some things just aren't worth it.

What do you think?

The Chakras

I was excited to find that Caroline Myss has a page of sacred essences for healing the chakras. She places monarda as resonating on chakra 5, the throat chakra. She speaks of how it stimulates communication. It reduces mucous and opens breathing.

I agree.

Stillpoint Aromatics, though, I feel are closer to being right.

They have it resonating on several;

Chakra 2 for relationships and creation energy

Chakra 4 for unconditional love

Chakra 6 for perspective, balancing and introspection. They list it as purifying and uplifting.

I feel all are correct. Certainly there is no tether in the base chakra, hence its lifting essence, and because it is so diffuse, floats right out of chakra 7 without even touching it...Up, up and away.

The Essential Oil

Tisserand and Young 2013 list Monarda as two oils

Monarda fistulosa L var menthaefolia as Wild Bergamot

Monarda didyma as Bee Balm

It seems likely that the name bee balm comes from its ability to soothe bee stings than being a plant attractive to bees. The petals are so tightly wound they are practically impossible for a bee to enter, instead being popular to butterflies and hummingbirds. *Didyma* has bright scarlet to magenta flowers.

The name *fistulosa* refers, again to the petals, meaning tubular

Typical Yield

0.65 to 1.2 g/100 g

Extraction

Steam distillation

Taxonomy

Lamiaceae

The copious planting of monarda is mainly due to the fact they are *gynodioecious*. This is often the case with plants from the lamiaceae genus. It means they have some plants where the flowers are all male and some that are female. Because the number of males flowers are far fewer the plant becomes functionally female and the male organs become sterile. Monarda acts, to all intents and purposes, like a hermaphrodite hence it is able to self-seed.

Main Producers

Canada (where some of the First Nations use the essential oil as well as the plant) and France.

Main constituents

Geraniol, Linalool, Thymol and Carvacrol as well as 1,8 cineole

Monarda is of great interest to the scientific community as they have tried to isolate a source of commercial geraniol, as it is showing anti-cancer effects, particularly in human colon cells. Most subspecies have been discounted with their high levels of thymol, but *Monarda fistulosa* constituents a massive 90% + of geraniol.

Effects of geraniol
- Found to be highly insecticidal

- Displays some anti-cancer effects

Effects of thymol

Highly antibacterial (used especially in mouthwashes)

- Cleanses of mucous

- Anti parasitic

- Relaxing to the uterus

Linalool

- Relaxing and distressing

- Leads to a decrease in aggressive behaviour

- Improves sleep

- Anti cancer, especially to liver cells

Carvacrol

- Protective, especially to the liver
- Anti bacterial
- Anti viral
- Reduces redness and swelling
- Supports blood sugar levels

1,8 cineole

- Respiratory
- Kill colds and viruses
- Analgesic

Blending Notes

Middle or heart note

Monarda fistulosa blends well with base notes such as sandalwood and benzoin, as well as floral notes like neroli and rose.

Monarda didyma blends with fresher more citrus-y notes like lemon and geranium.

Monarda in Clinical Trials

Insecticidal and anti-parasitic

Despite its long history of usage, surprisingly monarda seems not to have had much clinical investigation to day.

In Japan, in 2012, it was found to repel mosquitos but also to be antiplasmodial. Plasmodia is the parasite that causes malaria.

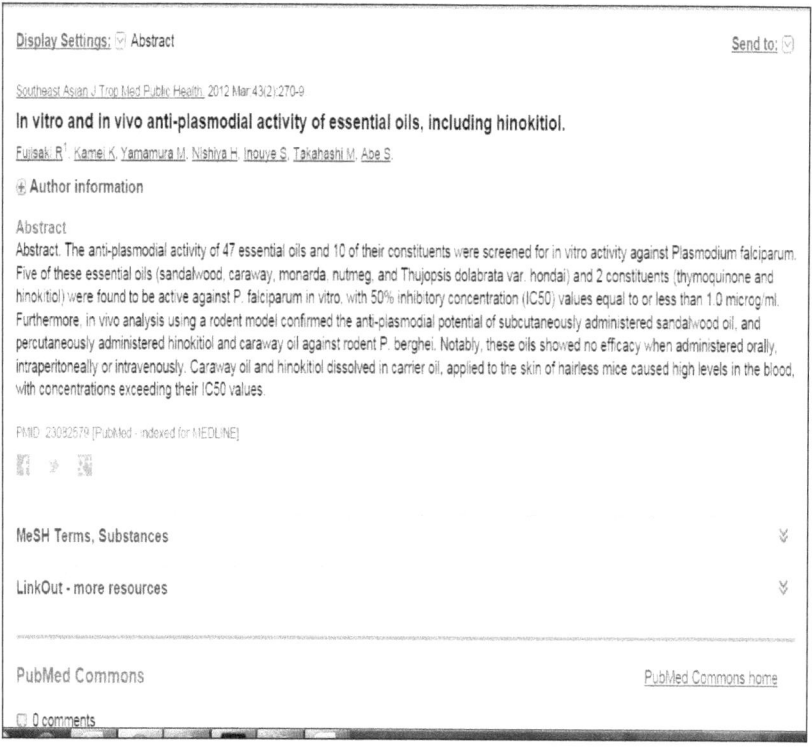

Display Settings: ☑ Abstract
Send to: ☑

Southeast Asian J Trop Med Public Health. 2012 Mar;43(2):270-9

In vitro and in vivo anti-plasmodial activity of essential oils, including hinokitiol.

Fujisaki R[1], Kamei K, Yamamura M, Nishiya H, Inouye S, Takahashi M, Abe S.

⊕ Author information

Abstract

Abstract. The anti-plasmodial activity of 47 essential oils and 10 of their constituents were screened for in vitro activity against Plasmodium falciparum. Five of these essential oils (sandalwood, caraway, monarda, nutmeg, and Thujopsis dolabrata var. hondai) and 2 constituents (thymoquinone and hinokitiol) were found to be active against P. falciparum in vitro, with 50% inhibitory concentration (IC50) values equal to or less than 1.0 microg/ml. Furthermore, in vivo analysis using a rodent model confirmed the anti-plasmodial potential of subcutaneously administered sandalwood oil, and percutaneously administered hinokitiol and caraway oil against rodent P. berghei. Notably, these oils showed no efficacy when administered orally, intraperitoneally or intravenously. Caraway oil and hinokitiol dissolved in carrier oil, applied to the skin of hairless mice caused high levels in the blood, with concentrations exceeding their IC50 values.

PMID: 23092579 [PubMed - indexed for MEDLINE]

MeSH Terms, Substances ⌄

LinkOut - more resources ⌄

PubMed Commons

PubMed Commons home

💬 0 comments

In 2009 Belgorod University in Russia declared it to be a more effective anti-seborrhoeic than using hydrocortisones because of its excellent anti-inflammatory effects

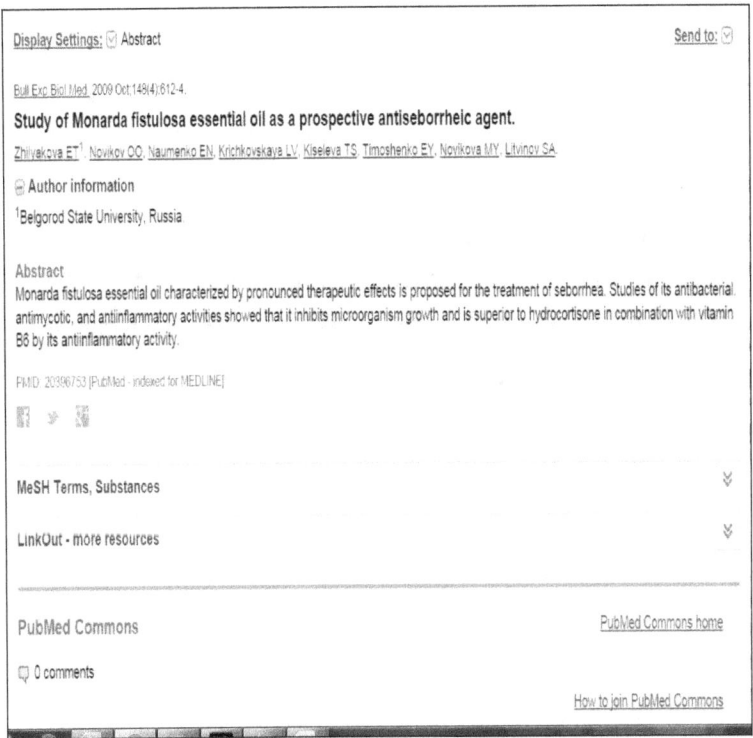

Bull Exp Biol Med. 2009 Oct;148(4):612-4.

Study of Monarda fistulosa essential oil as a prospective antiseborrheic agent.

Zhilyakova ET[1], Novikov OO, Naumenko EN, Krichkovskaya LV, Kiseleva TS, Timoshenko EY, Novikova MY, Litvinov SA.

Author information
[1]Belgorod State University, Russia

Abstract
Monarda fistulosa essential oil characterized by pronounced therapeutic effects is proposed for the treatment of seborrhea. Studies of its antibacterial, antimycotic, and antiinflammatory activities showed that it inhibits microorganism growth and is superior to hydrocortisone in combination with vitamin B6 by its antiinflammatory activity.

PMID: 20396753 [PubMed - indexed for MEDLINE]

Two other strains of monarda are tested. These are citriodora and puncta. I can find no references to either being commercially available as essential oils, but seeds for the plants seem to easy enough to find if you wanted to add them to your herb garden.

Monarda Citriodora

Amazingly this strand scored higher in anti-fungal efficacy than tea tree when tested on crops.

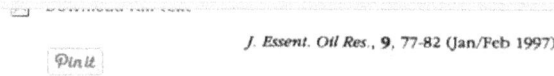

J. Essent. Oil Res., **9**, 77-82 (Jan/Feb 1997)

RESEARCH REPORT

Evaluation of the Antifungal Activity of the Essential Oils of *Monarda citriodora* var. *citriodora* and *Melaleuca alternifolia* on Post-Harvest Pathogens

Chris D. Bishop* and Ian B. Thornton
*School of Biological and Earth Sciences, Liverpool John Moores University
Byrom Street, Liverpool L3 3AF, UK*

Abstract

In vitro antifungal activity of the essential oils from *Monarda citriodora* and *Melaleuca alternifolia* was evaluated on 15 common post-harvest pathogens of a variety of crops. Both oils exhibited a high level of antifungal activity both by direct contact and in the vapor phase. Oil from *Monarda citriodora* was generally more active than that from *Melaleuca alternifolia*, particularly against more rapidly growing fungal species.

Key Word Index

Melaleuca alternifolia, Myrtaceae, tea-tree oil, *Monarda citriodora*, Labiatae, lemon bergamot, antifungal activity, post-harvest pathogens.

Introduction

Post-harvest disease caused by fungi is a major cause of product loss in many crops. The additional costs of harvest, transport and storage of produce mean that the economic cost of storage disease is proportionally higher than that caused by diseases in the field. Examination of the species causing wastage has shown that the same fungi, e.g. *Alternaria* spp., *Aspergillus* app., *Botrytis cinerea* Pers. and *Rhizopus* spp., are responsible in a wide range of different crops. Decay of fresh produce can be minimized by reducing mechanical damage through careful handling and also by storage under conditions that slow down senescence (1). These practices, however, are often insufficient to protect fungal invasion. Fungicide application is probably the most effective method of post-control (2). However, development of resistance to commonly used fungicides within

Citriodora has also been proven to have chemotherapeutic properties, causing cell death to cancer cells, in particular those of leukaemia

Display Settings: ⊙ Abstract

Send to: ⊙

Food Chem Toxicol. 2013 Dec:62:246-54. doi: 10.1016/j.fct.2013.08.037. Epub 2013 Aug 30

Disruption of the PI3K/AKT/mTOR signaling cascade and induction of apoptosis in HL-60 cells by an essential oil from Monarda citriodora.

Pathania AS[1], Guru SK, Verma MK, Sharma C, Abdullah ST, Malik F, Chandra S, Katoch M, Bhushan S.

⊕ Author information

Abstract

We have isolated an essential oil from Monarda citriodora (MC) and characterized its 22 chemical constituents with thymol (62%), carvacrol (4.82%), β-myrcene (3.45%), terpinen-4-ol (2.78%) and p-cymene (1.53%) representing the major constituents. We have reported for the first time the chemotherapeutic potential of MC in human promyelocytic leukemia HL-60 cells by means of apoptosis and disruption of the PI3K/AKT/mTOR signaling cascade. MC and its major constituent, thymol, inhibit the cell proliferation in different types of cancer cell lines like HL-60, MCF-7, PC-3, A-549 and MDAMB-231. MC was found to be more cytotoxic than thymol in HL-60 cells with an IC50 value of 22 μg/ml versus 45 μg/ml for thymol. Both MC and thymol induce apoptosis in HL-60 cells, which is evident by Hoechst staining, cell cycle analysis and immuno-expression of Bcl-xL, caspase-3,-8,-9 and PARP-1 cleavage. Both induce apoptosis by extrinsic and intrinsic apoptotic pathways that were confirmed by enhanced expression of death receptors (TNF-R1, Fas), caspase-9, loss of mitochondrial membrane potential and regression of Bcl-2/Bax ratio. Interestingly, both MC and thymol inhibit the downstream and upstream signaling of PI3K/AKT/mTOR pathway. The degree of apoptosis induction and disruption of the PI3K signaling cascade by MC was significantly higher when compared to thymol.

KEYWORDS: 3-(4,5-dimethylthiazole-2-yl)-2,5-diphenyl tetrazolium bromide; Apoptosis; Essential oil; FBS; MC; MTT; Monarda citriodora; PARP; PBS; PI; PI3K/AKT/mTOR; PTP; Rh-123; Rhodamine-123; VEGF; essential oil from Monarda citriodora; fetal bovine serum; mTOR; mammalian target of rapamycin; mitochondrial membrane potential; permeability transition pore; phosphate buffer saline; poly-ADP-ribose polymerase; propidium iodide; vascular endothelial growth factor; Δψmt

PMID: 23994707 [PubMed - in process]

Monarda punctata

Found to be anti-oxidant and to inhibit the streptococcus bacteria in the respiratory tract that causes membrane damage in chronic conditions such as bronchitis.

Display Settings: ⊙ Abstract

Send to: ⊙

Int J Clin Exp Pathol. 2014 Oct 15;7(11):7389-98. eCollection 2014

Antibacterial activity and mechanism of action of Monarda punctata essential oil and its main components against common bacterial pathogens in respiratory tract.

Li H[1], Yang T[1], Li FY[1], Yao Y[1], Sun ZM[1].

⊙ Author information

[1]Department of Respiratory and Critical Care Medicine, The First Affiliated Hospital of Xi'an Jiantong University Xi'an, China.

Abstract

The aim of the current research work was to study the chemical composition of the essential oil of Monarda punctata along with evaluating the essential oil and its major components for their antibacterial effects against some frequently encountered respiratory infection causing pathogens. Gas chromatographic mass spectrometric analysis revealed the presence of 13 chemical constituents with thymol (75.2%), p-cymene (6.7%), limonene (5.4), and carvacrol (3.5%) as the major constituents. The oil composition was dominated by the oxygenated monoterpenes. Antibacterial activity of the essential oil and its major constituents (thymol, p-cymene, limonene) was evaluated against Streptococcus pyogenes, methicillin-resistant Staphylococcus aureus (MRSA), Streptococcus pneumoniae, Haemophilus influenzae and Escherichia coli. The study revealed that the essential oil and its constituents exhibited a broad spectrum and variable degree of antibacterial activity against different strains. Among the tested strains, Streptococcus pyogenes, Escherichia coli and Streptococcus pneumoniae were the most susceptible bacterial strain showing lowest MIC and MBC values. Methicillin-resistant Staphylococcus aureus was the most resistant bacterial strain to the essential oil treatment showing relatively higher MIC and MBC values. Scanning electron microscopy revealed that the essential oil induced potent and dose-dependent membrane damage in S. pyogenes and MRSA bacterial strains. The reactive oxygen species generated by the Monarda punctata essential oil were identified using 2', 7'-dichlorofluorescein diacetate (DCFDA). This study indicated that the Monarda punctata essential oil to a great extent and thymol to a lower extent triggered a substantial increase in the ROS levels in S. pyogenes bacterial cultures which ultimately cause membrane damage as revealed by SEM results.

KEYWORDS: Monarda punctata; Streptococcus pyogenes; essential oil; methicillin-resistant Staphylococcus aureus; p-cymene; thymol

Growing Monarda

Monarda likes damp, disturbed soil. In full sun it can develop mildew and rusts.

It can be difficult to grow from seed. Easier, is to take cuttings in May- June. Cut off all but two leaves and cover entirely with compost in the winter.

There are many different colours of the flowers. Bear in mind that bees cannot distinguish reds and so are less likely to be attracted than if you plant lavender or purple shades.

It flowers between June and August. The flowers are fleeting, so deadhead regularly to lengthen its show. For distillation remove heads and leaves when about 80% open. Dry on racks or hanging up. Distil from dried matter.

Safety:

According to Tisserand and Young 2013 both essential oils of *Monarda fistulosa* and *didyma* hold the safety status of: *Generally Regarded As Safe*

Safe to use in pregnancy after 16 weeks.

High levels of geraniol mean it is a possible irritant to people who suffer from allergies to perfume.

Incidentally, according to some sources the ***herb*** (as opposed to the essential oil) is not suitable for use in pregnancy or on patients with thyroid problems.

Ways to administer Monarda Essential Oil

Creams and lotions

To my mind this is a super way to give an ongoing mega kick to bugs and viruses. Blend with eucalyptus, ravensara, tea tree or other anti virals to treat catarrh and chest infections

Massage Oils

Deliciously strengthening and soothing for little ones with coughs and colds

In the bath

Wallow in luxury, and I promise you nothing else really comes close to the relaxation of an aromatherapy bath. I tend not to make bath oils, rather a few drops straight in the water serves just as well.

Bye bye wretched day!

Diffusers

These have come a long way over the twenty years since I trained. Then you had to have a little candle under a warm bowl of water for the oils to diffuse. Now there are electronic gadgets to do the trick and they are ace.

Beautiful for meditation or helping you to sleep.

Candles

Beautiful, magickal, enigmatic.

Room sprays

These are a great way to clean your surroundings. If you don't like using chemical cleaning products, these are good to wipe down surfaces, telephones and light switches where dirt and germs like to breed.

Find yourself an atomiser spray. I use the ones you mist plants with. Use 12 drops of oil to a 50 ml bottle.

Now you can simply add the oils to distilled or tap water, but you will find the oils sink to the bottom. To break down the oils a little I add a teaspoon of vodka into the mix which also prevents oily stains on your lavender scented linen.

Bye bye bugs of the viral sort and the pesky winged variety too.

Steam Inhalations

Great for colds because it helps to unblock the sinuses, but I also do one of these once a week in my skin care regime to unblock the pores and really let the grime come away.

Any size bowl will do, but I use my pyrex apple crumble dish because it is big enough to get a good coverage of steam to my face but small enough to make a airtight tent with the towel!

Fill with boiling water, and add about 3 drops of essential oil.

KEEP A GOOD 6 - 8 INS AWAY FROM THE BOWL – any closer and you will scald your face.

Make a tent over your head with the towel so no steam can escape.

Compresses

There are two types of compresses, hot and cold. To choose which one to use, think about the effect you want to bring about. Heat will open up and release tissues, cold will cease and tighten them.

Hot compress

Fill the washing up bowl with just warmer than hand hot water and then add 5 drops of essential oil. Soak your compress and wring out well. Place on the affected part, and keep warm with a hot water bottle on top. Leave for 5 mins

What is important to remember is when you draw toxins out into a compress, it brings body salts with it. These are very corrosive to towels!! Don't throw your towel in the laundry basket and forget about it because when you come to wash it...it will be full of holes! Wash out compresses immediately. Many people use pieces of muslin, I just use an old towel.

Monarda Recipes

Those who read more of my work will probably smile, knowing how much I hate writing recipes. The very nature of healing is it is individual to each patient. The reasons for the illness are diverse and so therefore are the blends to create them. Since people keep asking me for them, though, I am here to please.

Please don't use this as the *be-all-and-end- all* of your use of your new bottle of oil. Download The Complete Guide of Clinical Aromatherapy and The Essential Oils of The Physical Body, to get far more respiratory, soothing and stomachic oils to blend with it. Use The Essential of The Mind Body Spirit to tap into more emotional aspects of using it for healing.

Please, be creative, be innovative and be your very *own* brand of healer.

Baby Chest Infection Lotion

100 ml / 4 oz blank lotion or massage oil

Monarda x 1

Benzoin x 1

Camomile x 1

Massage lightly onto baby's back to open the airways and relieve catarrh.

Breathe Easy Bath
Run a warm bath and add

Monarda x 2

Myrtle x 3

Eucalypus globulus x 3

Colic compress
Monarda x 1

Carrot x 1

Dill x 1

Fill washing up bowl with warm water, then add these oils. Soak a flannel and place on baby's tummy. Ensure she stays warm. Compresses can make temperatures drop quickly. (Also, of course, that is one of monarda's properties)

Oily Skin Toner

Lavender x 1

Neroli x 1

Monarda x 2

Meditation to let go of the past

Monarda x 2

Geranium x 1

Rose x 1

(See The Essential Oils of The Mind Body Spirit for more specific oils choices to substitute with rose i.e for jealousy – *ylang ylang*, *vetiver* for long hidden secrets etc)

Chakra Mediations

There are many ways to meditate, but for the purposes of this book we shall focus on vitalising and balancing the chakras.

You will often see people meditating sitting in the lotus position, so they have contact with the root chakra and the floor. It is not necessary to sit cross legged, you can achieve the same objective sitting upright in a chair or lying on your back on the bed.

Close your eyes and breathe slowly and deliberately. We want to build the breathing up in cycles where we breathe in for four and out for eight. This is the cycle used in transcendental meditation and has been proven to be the best way to release endorphins in the brain, which of course is useful for pain relief.

Once you have mastered the breathing pattern, see a white light coming out of your head, like a fountain and coming down the side of your body, completely surrounding it. Let the light do this six times so you are entirely surrounded and completely protected by it. We call this psychically protecting ourselves. This is vital and you must do this every time you meditate (and everytime you heal or massage someone).

Now we are going to focus on the chakras and we want to see them start to pulsate open and closed, regularly, rhythmically and brightly.

First, see a violet light above your head.

Then when you are happy it is bright and energetic, move your focus to the brow and visualise a deep rich indigo there.

At the throat, see blue.

The heart, green.

Yellow at the solar plexus

Orange at the abdomen

Red at the root

Now, remember that monarda has no grounding mechanism so really focus on anchoring red.

Then when you are happy they are nourished and vital, repeat the white light fountain six more complete times around you.

Lastly imagine a beautiful golden rain, cleansing your white bubble, washing away any germs, impurities or negative energy you may have collected.

Open your eyes.

Monarda Blends for Chakra Meditation

Chakra 1

Not indicated as having any action

Blend for chakra 2

Cardamom x 1

Jasmine x 1

Monarda x 1

Blend for chakra 3

Rose x 1

Neroli x 1

Monarda x 1

Blend for Chakra 4

Orange x 1

Basil x 1

Monarda x 3

Blend for Chakra 5

Helichrysm x 2

Cedarwood x 1

Monarda x 3

Blend for Chakra 6

Black pepper x 1

Rose otto x 1

Monarda x 2

Chakra 7

Not indicated as having any actions

Colour Vibration

Blue

Musical Vibration

Monarda vibrates in the chord of F Major, so it has a bright happy resonance (this is the key of the English Horn) it is a very deliberate and determined key. Incidentally, it is one of the most difficult chords for guitarists to play. It is complex and is seen a bit like the musical Holy Grail. It requires effort and you will see in the song choices, this translates into the songs written around it. Meditating with music in the same key helps to draw more senses into the treatment, making it an even more powerful therapy.

A relaxing classical piece you might consider is Water Music Suite No.1 for Orchestra by Handel, or JS Bach's Brandenburg Concertos Numbers 1 & 2.

If you are infusing to get some serious happy vibes going on: Madonna's *Open Your Heart*, Natasha Beddingfield's *Unwritten* and Diana Ross's *I'm Coming Out*. Of course, what we are striving for here is more and more novel ways to get better and in praise of that let's scream "You ain't seen the best of me..." with Irene Cara's *Fame*.

For nights when you are working hard to break the emotional ties, I am not sure you could ever beat Gary Moore's, *I Still Got The Blues For You* (now he really can play in F major. That's some serious guitar playing!) or Bill Wither's *Ain't No Sunshine Now She's Gone*.

Something a bit heavier? Red Hot Chilli Peppers *Scar Tissue*, Avril Lavigne *Complicated, Hand of Doom* by Black Sabbath and Paramour's *Future*.

Simply google songs written in F Major to create your own monarda play list.

Prayer of Gratitude

And finally, it seems only fitting that our prayers of gratitude be from the plains where our knowledge of monarda originated.

Native American Prayer

Great Spirit,
Give us hearts to understand
Never to take from creation's beauty more
than we give,
Never to destroy want only for the furtherance
of greed,
Never to deny to give our hands for the
building of earth's beauty,
Never to take from her what we cannot use.

Give us hearts to understand
That to destroy earth's music is to create
confusion,
That to wreck her appearance is to blind us to
beauty,
That to callously pollute her fragrance is to
make a house of stench,
That as we care for her she will care for us.

Give us hearts to understand
We have forgotten who we are.
We have sought only our own security.
We have exploited simply for our own ends.
We have distorted our knowledge.
We have abused our power.

Great Spirit,
Whose dry lands thirst,
Help us to find the way to refresh your lands.

Great Spirit,
Whose waters are choked with debris and
pollution,
Help us to find the way to cleanse your waters.

Great Spirit,
Whose beautiful earth grows ugly with
misuse,
Help us to find the way to restore beauty to
your handiwork.

Great Spirit,
Whose creatures are being destroyed,

Help us to find a way to replenish them

Great Spirit,
whose gifts to us are being lost in selfishness
and corruption,
Help us to find the way to restore our
humanity.

~Author Unknown

Authors comment.

In my book The Aromatherapy Bronchitis Treatment, I speak of how monarda can help a complication of COPD for wound healing. The book in its entirety is about how holding onto certain negative emotions can lead to inflammation. Monarda oil seems to hold up a mirror to the research and say physical healing or emotional? For many generations to come yet, I fear we will not be able to say.

Plants though, are enigmatic things and their consciousness makes them change, evolve and adapt to meet the requirements of their surroundings. In a 2011 paper *Survival of three commercially available natural enemies exposed to Michigan wildflowers*, a description was given of how monarda changed in physical appearance, but also how the very physiology of the plant changed when it was placed by other wild flowers. Scientific proof then that Monarda can adapt, as every other plant can, to the environment she finds herself in.

In her book The Garden of Eden, Jill Bruce writes:

> *As arrogant humans, we assume the Earth is run on scientific lines, and we are in charge.*
>
> *Not completely so.*

When I wrote the first edition of this book, way back in 1992, I was startled to find that plants evolve. They have 'aerials' into our world, from which they receive knowledge to make medicines for us, way before we think we need them.

That made me think...

Monarda was introduced to Britain in 1637. Tobacco had been previously been bought to England in 1564. When I asked about UK awareness of Monarda oil on facbook.com/TheSecretHealerWrites, it was very small, and there are some extremely experienced aromatherapists hanging out there. And yet, it is sold on many suppliers sites.

UK women are facing their biggest health crisis to date, COPD. Now far outstripping the number of women who die from cancer or coronary heart disease (and in fact, outstripping the number of men too!) respiratory disease is severely bad news.

And then here, seemingly out of nowhere, mentioned very little in British texts, comes a medicine from the very people who first introduced us to tobacco.

More than that too, the Elk Medicine seems to be revealing herself at a time when consciousness is very much moving towards the feminine. Of empowerment of women, alone, but even more so in groups....Again, this is a very new a powerful change in the consciousness of Britain as a whole.

Collect, group, sort, organise, these are the emotions of Monarda

These are also, I hope, what you will want to do with the oils profiles I have written!

The plan was initially to try to publish one a week but they are so much more complex than I thought they would be, it looks like they will come out two a fortnight, Whether I can sustain that alongside my medical research remains to be seen. I hope so because they are fascinating to write.

In tend to dedicate each of these profiles to a different fan on facbook.com/TheSecretHealerWrites to recognise how much appreciate the collaborations and efforts people put in supporting my work, commenting, liking and sharing. This first one goes to Clare of Clare Ella Aromatherapy who has a practice in Lincoln and is quite honestly the hardest working, bravest and most dedicated therapist I know.

Clare: I am honoured to call you my friend and I cannot thank you for everything you do.

Please reader, if you would, leave me a review about this book. I cannot tell you how much they help, but they also really make me smile. I do read them all, and I try to reply. If you do want to get in contact with me, I spend an unhealthy amount of time on facebook! You can contact me at facbook.com/TheSecretHealerWrites and I will happily try to answer any questions for you, if I know how.

Most useful to me, would be if you could post some suggestions of oils you would like to know more about. I get very bored trying to think up ideas!!!

Before I go, I would also like to suggest you try reading George Shepherd's profiles too. They are very good and I completely stole the idea of copying the trial papers into the documents from him, so I kinda owe him! His works tend to be on more widely used oils than mine, I think because he seem more interested in focusing on the clinical trials. Collecting these will really help to grow the information in your files.

Review and Buy!! Bye!

Liz

Post script: Plant medicine is my life, and I know a great deal about it. Native American life and culture, however, is not my world. I have tried my best to offer due respect to the peoples whose medicine this is. There has been a great deal of effort to use the politically correct terminology for each nation and their past. If I have made any errors, please can I apologise for my ignorance; most certainly no offence is intended.

Other books in The Secret Healer Series

The Essential Oils Profiles

Vetiver

Coming soon....

Basil

Cedarwood

Sandalwood

Patchouli

To get the very best from your learning experience, why not treat yourself to one of the Secret Healer Training Manuals? To begin with, have you taken advantage of the free essential oil profiles available in...

Book 1 - The Complete Guide to

Clinical Aromatherapy & Essential Oils for the Physical Body

Essentially...essential oils for beginners, talented novices and intermediate aromatherapists

Let me ask you, why do you want a book on aromatherapy?

Do you want to learn how to care for your family naturally?

Perhaps you have a franchise selling essential oils and want to know more about what they can do?

Maybe you love the delicious scents and want understand how these beautiful things come to heal.

I wonder if you have started to learn and now want to discover how to build on your knowledge.

Whatever you are looking for this book has something for you.

- Details of how to treat over 60 conditions with essential oils
- Profiles of over 100 natural plant essences and their safety data
- Descriptions of 15 carrier oils and their applications not only for massage but also adding to creams and lotions.
- Comprehensive data of how the chemistry of an oil will affect its actions
- In depth insights into how professional aromatherapists blend...including their 13 favourite recipes from their practices.

Including....

- Sensuous aromatherapy blends by a qualified sex therapist
- Two blends for labour by the midwife running an aromatherapy program on an NHS maternity ward
- A blend for depression by a qualified mental health

PLUS....

10 bonus essential oil monographs and a complementary hypnotherapy relaxation download.

Discount vouchers of treatments courses and products by participating therapists.

AND.... for those of you who would like to contribute, there is a chance to make a donation to cancer research too.

This is my gift to you.

Download for FREE - From 30.11.14

Book 2 Essential Oils for Mind Body Spirit

The Holistic Medicine of Clinical Aromatherapy

Healing the skin, easing the tummy ache or getting someone to sleep is easy with essential oils. Anyone can do it. The joy of healing, though, comes from peeling back the layers of the disease, almost like a detective to find out exactly what caused it in the first place.

Consider this book to be lesson 2 in The Secret Healer Series.

You have mastered which oil to use for what and why...this book takes you step by step though the ancient healing mechanisms of the aura, the chakras and meridians but also explores how that ties in with the latest scientific discoveries into how the emotions affect our health. Using Candace Pert's remarkable "Molecules of Emotion" research, The Secret Healer shows you *where* to look for healing links and *why*.

- Uncover how a certain recurrent negative emotion can be the trigger to make you ill?
- Understand internal processes that mean that psychology, neurology and immunology are quintessentially, and inextricably linked.
- Learn how to use essential oils control your emotions and in turn bring about a far greater standard of wellness.
- Discover mindblowing research that shows the emotions we experience are actually the sensations of neuropeptides triggering our organs to do their jobs
- Reflect on the wonder of Chinese medicine and ancient healing being completely accurate in their healing

mechanisms for thousands of years...now that science proves it to be so.

Essential Oils for The Mind Body Spirit couples ancient wisdom with cutting edge science. This is the knowledge the drug companies hope you never find out and our doctors pray we all will.

A short write up, for a book that will change your life. I promise you, when you read the latest findings of psychoneuroimmunology, you will never waste another day on being angry again.

Book 3 The Essential Oil Liver Cleanse
The Professional Aromatherapist's Liver Detox

We are warned of the threats of heart attacks, strokes and cancer, especially if we are overweight.

What is kept quieter is doctors have established a link between toxicity in the liver and metabolic syndrome, the condition that leads to many of these conditions. What's more non fatty liver disease is known to underlie many other conditions such as eczema, allergies and headaches.

The scandal is just how many of our livers are struggling under the strain of over processed foods, pharmaceutical debris and actually even our own bad tempers!

This book explains:

- The importance of the liver and its functions
- How it becomes dysfunctional and how to interpret warning signposts
- How to cleanse and nourish using not just essential oils, but also vitamins and minerals and diet.
- The strange correlation between how our emotions translate negativity into disease.
- How to implement other therapies such as chiropractic, acupressure and counselling and how to secure fantastic referrals.

This book is best used in tandem with The Professional Stress Solution to benefit from the complementary healing. Use Sales Strategies for Gentle Souls to create a marketing plan to use your new found knowledge to smash your competition out of the water!!!

Book 4 The Professional Stress Solution

Essential Oils and Holistic Health Stress Management Techniques for The Professional Aromatherapist

Stress is pandemic in our society.

Scientists agree it plays a quintessential role in how likely it is we will suffer from chronic and possibly fatal illnesses in the future. Risk factors of metabolic syndrome, diabetes, stroke and heart disease are increased through stress.

The daft thing is....aromatherapy can do amazing things to ease it, and potentially aromatherapists could take a massive workload away from the doctors' surgeries.

- Discover the hormonal changes and peptide triggers that change a person's health and mental state.
- Learn how it affects the liver, adrenals and pituitary gland.
- Uncover the strange phenomenon of Yin disease
- Build a better foundation of care, but also a knowledge base that means you can sell your treatments more effectively.
- Improve your healing skills set
- Supercharge your referrals potential from other complementary therapists and orthodox medicine alike.

Includes free bonus material of

- Chiropractic chart of misalignments and potential organic disturbance
- Chart of the meridians and suggested acupressure points to detox the organs more quickly
- Detailed information about how to improve the patients condition with vitamin and minerals therapy
- In depth dietary advice
- Free hypnotherapy relaxation download

Essential Oils are The Off Switch for stress. The *Professional Stress Solution* is the ON SWITCH for your aromatherapy business.

Book 5 The Aromatherapy Eczema Treatment

Healing Eczema, Itchy Skin Rashes and Atopic Dermatitis with Essential Oils and Holistic Medicine

Most people appreciate that the itching and redness of eczema can be used using essential oils, but what if I told you they were capable of so much more?

Imagine if, as a therapist, you were able to pinpoint the emotions that set off these flares? Can you visualise what it would mean to your patient if you were able to isolate the very protagonist causing the eczema breakout and alleviate their pain completely?

Well now you can.

This book teaches you:

- How to isolate the emotions causing the emotional cycle of pain
- The likely food triggers for your patient and the tools to identify the exact times they will detonate a reaction
- The familial traits and links that lead to atopic eczema
- How these links connect with the liver and in turn how to cleanse the liver toxicity
- Vitamins and minerals to cleanse and nourish the system

The book contains very real that will not only transform the way you treat clients, but will skyrocket your clinic's takings.

I recommend reading this book in tandem with *The Professional Stress Solution* and the *Essential Oil Liver Cleanse* to fully understand the cycles and processes of treatment. Add to it *Sales Strategies for Gentle Souls* and your business will stand on an entirely new footing.

Why not save yourself 1/3

And treat yourself to the set?

The full and comprehensive course into how to heal eczema

with aromatherapy and essential oils **$9.99 / £5.99**

The Aromatherapy Bronchitis Treatment

Support the Respiratory System with Essential Oils and Holistic Medicine for COPD, Emphysema, Acute and Chronic Bronchitis Symptoms

Breathing is the most natural thing in the world. It *should* be effortless, free and easy.
But if you are reading this...the chances are *your* breathing is not.

You are not alone. In fact COPD is **now the second biggest cause of death in the UK and the third in the United States**. Respiratory disease is seriously bad news. Placing a massive burden on healthcare provision, **doctors place self care for respiratory disorders as one of their highest priorities**.

The question is...where on earth does one start?

Well, interestingly in these days of drug resistant bugs and infections, scientists are exploring respiratory medicine through a whole new realm...that of the plant kingdom. Over and over again they are finding that essential oils offer some of the best effects for bronchitis, emphysema and COPD.

Moreover, the scholars of psychoneuroimmunology have now concluded that the emotions (particularly from the past) play a vital role in the body's propensity to develop COPD, and that stress and hostility will assuredly make symptoms worse.

Together with detailed investigations into the essential oils to help maintain and support a healthy respiratory system, we look at how diet, emotional wellness and lifestyle changes can break the cycle of respiratory disease.

Some oils you may be able to guess; others are so unexpected they are like a bolt from the blue!

Discover:

- The essential oils found to be the most effective in **reducing inflammation, mucous and pain.**
- The hazardous oil able to positively affect Nitric Oxide, the gas considered vital to cardio vascular health and successful respiratory health.
- The foods suggested by doctors and nutritionists **to break the cycle of disease and support a healthier respiratory system**
- **Safe and clear instructions** on how to use which oil and when.
- Aromatherapy recipes to **clear infection, reduce pain, ease breathing and calm coughing.**

Sick of being sick...?

Relax...*breathe....we've got this covered.*

Improve your breathing, your sleep, even your emotional state and take the first steps on the road to getting your life back.

Clear, simple to follow advice and insights into your illness I'll bet you never even considered before!

Sales Strategies for Gentle Souls

Targeted Sales Training for Professional Aromatherapists

Wonderful things are happening in complementary therapy. Very gifted people are churning out fantastic research and results. The internet is full of what essential oils can do. But when a gentle soul emerges from their relaxing haze of their aromatherapy class room, how do they harness the buzz of energy around them for their craft?

From 1999-2008 I worked in one of the most aggressive commercial environments there is. My role as a recruitment consultant was 80% cold calling in an extremely saturated sales arena. Despite my own gentle soul, I found ways not only to compete, but to excel.

- Learn how to pinpoint the best customers for your practice
- Cost your treatments to ensure every treatment is profitable for both you and your customer
- Discover how to make every conversation into a potential sale lead without becoming a complete and utter pain in the a*s!
- Uncover the reasons why you are not closing sales so you never have to make the same mistakes again
- Create a growth environment where you plan success and always find yourself stepping into it

If you are working with essential oils, and you want to make a good living for it, then you need to learn to sell. What's more, if you are going to say "selling doesn't work on my customers"....then you have simply been taught to do it wrongly.

My dream is to see aromatherapy at the forefront of medicine. I need an army of gifted healers to achieve that. Consider yourself to be my newest recruit and I am going to drill you till you are the slickest, subtlest and most effective marketeer there is. You have the knowledge to make people better, now let me give you the business prowess to heal even more people than you have ever done before.

The Secret Healer has stress in her sights and she's about to make a killing. Listen carefully...she has much to tell you. £1.99 / $2.99

Buy now

www.thesecrethealer.co.uk

www.buildyourownreality.com

About the Author

Elizabeth Ashley qualified as an aromatherapist in 1993, and then passed her Advanced Aromatherapy Diploma in 1994. She has been practicing aromatherapy for almost 21 years.

In 1999, she fell into a whole new career in the aggressive commercial sector of recruitment consultancy. There she discovered her father's second hand car salesman genes had passed along and found she had quite a gift of the gab! More than that, she discovered she could sell...and then some.

In 2008, Elizabeth fell ill during pregnancy with a blood clot in her lungs. The pulmonary embolism prevented her from working and she started to write. Very quickly she gained her first contract as a ghost writer...a recipe book for cheese cakes!

In 2010 she was published professionally for her work on Galbanum oil in the Aromatherapy Thymes, journal of the International Federation of Aromatherapists, and on Tuberose oil by the New Zealand Register of Holistic Therapist.

In 2011 she was seconded on a consultative basis to Walsall Independent Treatment Centre, designed to be a rainbow bridge between traditional and complementary medicines. There she became aware of the rumblings of change in healthcare. Her book *Sales Strategies for Gentle Souls* explains the connotations of this.

Many of her books are aimed at helping qualified aromatherapists to expand their healing repertoire and build their businesses. She also writes for people who have an interest in essential oils and want to learn how to heal. Her in depth essential oil profiles chart the healing properties of plants from the most arcane depths of historic folklore up to the scientific lab trials of today.

In 2014 she ranks in the top 50 contract writers on the freelancer marketplace Elance.com. She is the ghost writer of seven number one Amazon best sellers in the natural healing category. She lives in Shropshire with her husband and youngest son, kept company by their cat, the budgie and many shoals of tropical fish! Her elder son and daughter attend University and make her prouder than anything ever could.

Elizabeth Ashley is possibly one of the most published aromatherapy writers you have never heard of! By 2015, all of that will have changed. Elizabeth Ashley is *The Secret Healer*.

Works Cited

Beauchamp, A. (2013, 07 15). *Wild Bergamot - Monarda Fistulosa*. Retrieved 02 04, 2015, from Dharani Healing Arts: http://www.dharanihealingarts.com/wild-bergamot-monarda-fistulosa/

Deep Glade Apothecary. (2012, 04 03). *Wild Bee Balm, Monarda Fistulosa*. Retrieved 02 03, 2015, from Natures Alive: https://naturesalive.wordpress.com/2012/04/03/wild-bee-balm-monarda-fistulosa/

Diamon, A. C. (Not found). *Individual plant essences*. Retrieved 01 03, 2015, from Diamon Naturals: http://www.diamon-naturals.us/individualFE.htm

Elland, S. (2008). *Monarda Fistulosa*. Retrieved 02 04, 2015, from Plant Lives: http://www.plantlives.com/docs/M/Monarda_fistulosa.pdf

Emory Dean Keoke, K. M. (2001). *Encyclopaedia of American Indians Contrtibutions to the World*. Facts on File Inc.

Esther Bailón-García *, F. J.-H.-C. (2013). *Catalysts Supported on Carbon Materials for the Selective*. Retrieved 02 04, 2015, from Mdpi.com: file:///C:/Users/Home/Downloads/catalysts-03-00853.pdf

Fragrant Earth. (Unlisted). *Monarda Bee Balm Essential Oil.* Retrieved 02 05, 2015, from Fragrant Earth: http://www.stillpointaromatics.com/monarda-fistulosa-wild-bergamot-essential-oil-aromatherapy

G. Mazza, B. B. (n.d.). *Essential oil of Monardafistulosa L. var. Menthaefolia, a potential source of geraniol.* Retrieved 02 2015, 05, from Researchgate: http://www.researchgate.net/publication/230087351_Essenti al_oil_of_Monardafistulosa_L._var._Menthaefolia_a_potent ial_source_of_geraniol

G. Mazza, F. K. (1993). *Monarda: A Source of Geraniol, Linalool, Thymol and Carvacrol-rich Essential Oils.* Retrieved 02 05, 2015, from Horticulture and Landscape Architecture|Purdue University: https://www.hort.purdue.edu/newcrop/proceedings1993/v2-628.html

Kress, H. (Unlisted). *Monarda.* Retrieved 02 05, 2015, from Hernritettes Herb: http://www.henriettes-herb.com/eclectic/kings/monarda.html

Lag., C. e. (2012). *Monarda Citriodora.* Retrieved 02 04, 2015, from Plants for A Future: http://www.pfaf.org/user/Plant.aspx?LatinName=Monarda+citriodora

M, S. K. (n.d.). *Wild Beramot; Monarda Fistulosa*. Retrieved from Tumblr: http://silverknightm.tumblr.com/post/84099855123/bergam ot-wild-monarda-fistulosa-folk-names

Mariko Namba Walter, E. J. (2004). *Shamanism: An Encyclopedia of World Beliefs, Practices, and Culture, Volume 1*. ABC-CLIO Ltd.

Myss, C. (Copyright 2015). *Sacred Chakra Oils Set*. Retrieved 02 03, 2015, from Myss.com: http://www.myss.com/catalog/sacred-chakra-oils-set.htm

Pepper, D. (2008-2015). *Purple Monarda Flower Essence* . Retrieved 02 03, 2015, from Tree Frog Farm: http://www.treefrogfarm.com/store/flower-essences-tree-essences/purple-monarda-flower-essence.html

Pepper, J. a. (Unlisted). *Purple Monarda Flower Essence*. Retrieved 02 05, 2015, from Tree Frog Farm: http://www.treefrogfarm.com/store/flower-essences-tree-essences/purple-monarda-flower-essence.html

Rohlfson, W. (2014, 09 08). *Patent: Method for Cultivation of Monarda Fistulosa for Production of Thymoquinone*. Retrieved 02 05, 2015, from Google Patents: http://www.google.com/patents/US20140275585

Rosa, K. (2006, 10). *Mountain Majesty.* Retrieved 02 04, 2015, from Desert Exposure: http://www.desertexposure.com/200610/200610_bms_mountain_monarda.html

Rose, K. (2006, 02 07). *Monarda.* Retrieved 02 04, 2015, from The Medicine Woamn's Roots: http://bearmedicineherbals.com/monarda.html

Rose, K. (2009). *The Enchantment of Bee Balm.* Retrieved 02 03, 2015, from Bear Medicine Herbals : http://bearmedicineherbals.com/flowers-from-the-faerygrounds-the-enchantment-of-beebalm.html

Roth, H. A. (2006). *Monarda Fistulosa; Wild Bergamot.* Retrieved 02 04, 2015, from Alchemy Works: http://www.alchemy-works.com/monarda_fistulosa.html

Smal, E. *North American Cornucopia: Top 100 Indigenous Food Plants.* CRC Press.

Still Point Aromatics. (2014). *Monarda Fistulosa Essential Oil.* Retrieved 02 04, 2015, from Still Point Aromatics: http://www.stillpointaromatics.com/monarda-fistulosa-wild-bergamot-essential-oil-aromatherapy

Tabanca N1, B. U. (2013). *Bioassay-guided investigation of two Monarda essential oils as repellents of yellow fever mosquito Aedes aegypti*. Retrieved 02 03, 2013, from Pubmed: http://www.ncbi.nlm.nih.gov/pubmed/23919579

Tabanca N1, B. U. (2013, 09). *Bioassay-guided investigation of two Monarda essential oils as repellents of yellow fever mosquito Aedes aegypti*. Retrieved 02 04, 2015, from Pubmed: http://www.ncbi.nlm.nih.gov/pubmed/23919579

TeiF, T. (2011). *Bee Balm aka Monarda Essential Oil, Organically Grown in Ontario!* Retrieved 02 15, 2015, from Anarres Health: http://www.anarreshealth.ca/node/1717

The Aroma Alternatives Limited. (Unlisted). *Monarda Essential Oil*. Retrieved 02 04, 2015, from Ingredients to Die For:
http://www.ingredientstodiefor.com/item/Monarda_Essential_Oil_/1254

The Southwest School of Botanical Medicine. (1912). *Uses of Plants by the Indians of the Missouri River Region* . Retrieved 02 04, 2015, from South West School of Botanical Medicine: http://www.swsbm.com/Ethnobotany/MissouriValley-Gilmore-1.pdf

Thorntona, C. D. (1977). *Evaluation of the Antifungal Activity of the Essential Oils of Monarda citriodora var. citriodora and Melaleuca alternifolia on Post-Harvest Pathogens*. Retrieved 02 03, 2015, from Taylor and Francis Online:

http://www.tandfonline.com/doi/abs/10.1080/10412905.199
7.9700718#.VNCxf8msXUI

Walter, J. (1919). *Designs_on_Prehistoric_Hopi_Pottery*.
Retrieved 02 04, 2015, from Forgotten Books:
http://www.forgottenbooks.com/readbook_text/Designs_on
_Prehistoric_Hopi_Pottery_1000764718/145

Witchipedia. (n.d.). *Monarda*. Retrieved 02 04, 2015, from
Witchipedia: http://www.witchipedia.com/herb:monarda

Wood, M. (1997). *The Book of Herbal Wisdom: Using Plants
as Medicine*. North Atlantic Books.

Wrencsh, R. (1992). *The Essence of Herbs* . University Press of
Missisippi .

Zhan Guo Lu, X. H. (2011, 01). *Chemical Composition of
Antibacterial Activity of Essential Oil from Monarda
citriodora Flowers*. Retrieved 02 04, 2015, from Scientific.
net: http://www.scientific.net/AMR.183-185.920

Zhilyakova ET1, N. O. (2009). *Study of Monarda fistulosa
essential oil as a prospective antiseborrheic agent*. Retrieved
02 03, 2015, from Pubmed:
http://www.ncbi.nlm.nih.gov/pubmed/20396753

Disclaimer

by SEQ Legal

(1)   Introduction

This disclaimer governs the use of this book. [By using this book, you accept this disclaimer in full. / We will ask you to agree to this disclaimer before you can access the book.]

(2)   Credit

This disclaimer was created using an <u>SEQ Legal</u> template.

(3)   No advice

The book contains information about aromatherapy and the use of essential oils.The information is not advice, and should not be treated as such.

[You must not rely on the information in the book as an alternative to qualified medical advice from a health professional. advice from an appropriately qualified professional. If you have any specific questions about any medical matter you should consult an appropriately qualified professional.]

[If you think you may be suffering from any medical condition you should seek immediate medical attention. You should never delay seeking medical advice, disregard medical advice, or discontinue medical treatment because of information in the book.]

(4) No representations or warranties

To the maximum extent permitted by applicable law and subject to section 6 below, we exclude all representations, warranties, undertakings and guarantees relating to the book.

Without prejudice to the generality of the foregoing paragraph, we do not represent, warrant, undertake or guarantee:

> that the information in the book is correct, accurate, complete or non-misleading;

> that the use of the guidance in the book will lead to any particular outcome or result; or

> in particular, that by using the guidance in the book you will heal disease or work in any way as a cure for illness.

(5)   Limitations and exclusions of liability

The limitations and exclusions of liability set out in this section and elsewhere in this disclaimer: are subject to section 6 below; and govern all liabilities arising under the disclaimer or in relation to the book, including liabilities arising in contract, in tort (including negligence) and for breach of statutory duty.

We will not be liable to you in respect of any losses arising out of any event or events beyond our reasonable control.

We will not be liable to you in respect of any business losses, including without limitation loss of or damage to profits, income, revenue, use, production, anticipated savings, business, contracts, commercial opportunities or goodwill.

We will not be liable to you in respect of any loss or corruption of any data, database or software.

We will not be liable to you in respect of any special, indirect or consequential loss or damage.

(6)   Exceptions

Nothing in this disclaimer shall: limit or exclude our liability for death or personal injury resulting from negligence; limit or exclude our liability for fraud or fraudulent misrepresentation; limit any of our liabilities in any way that is not permitted under applicable law; or exclude any of our liabilities that may not be excluded under applicable law.

(7)   Severability

If a section of this disclaimer is determined by any court or other competent authority to be unlawful and/or unenforceable, the other sections of this disclaimer continue in effect.

If any unlawful and/or unenforceable section would be lawful or enforceable if part of it were deleted, that part will be deemed to be deleted, and the rest of the section will continue in effect.

(8)   Law and jurisdiction

This disclaimer will be governed by and construed in accordance with English law, and any disputes relating to this disclaimer will be subject to the exclusive jurisdiction of the courts of England and Wales.

(9)   Our details

In this disclaimer, "we" means (and "us" and "our" refer to) *Build Your Own Reality.com* of *SY8 1LQ*.